I am not a Doctor or specialist and this is not a diet. This is my story on how I lost 100 pounds and kept it off without surgery. People asked me "how I did it?" and this is how I did it.

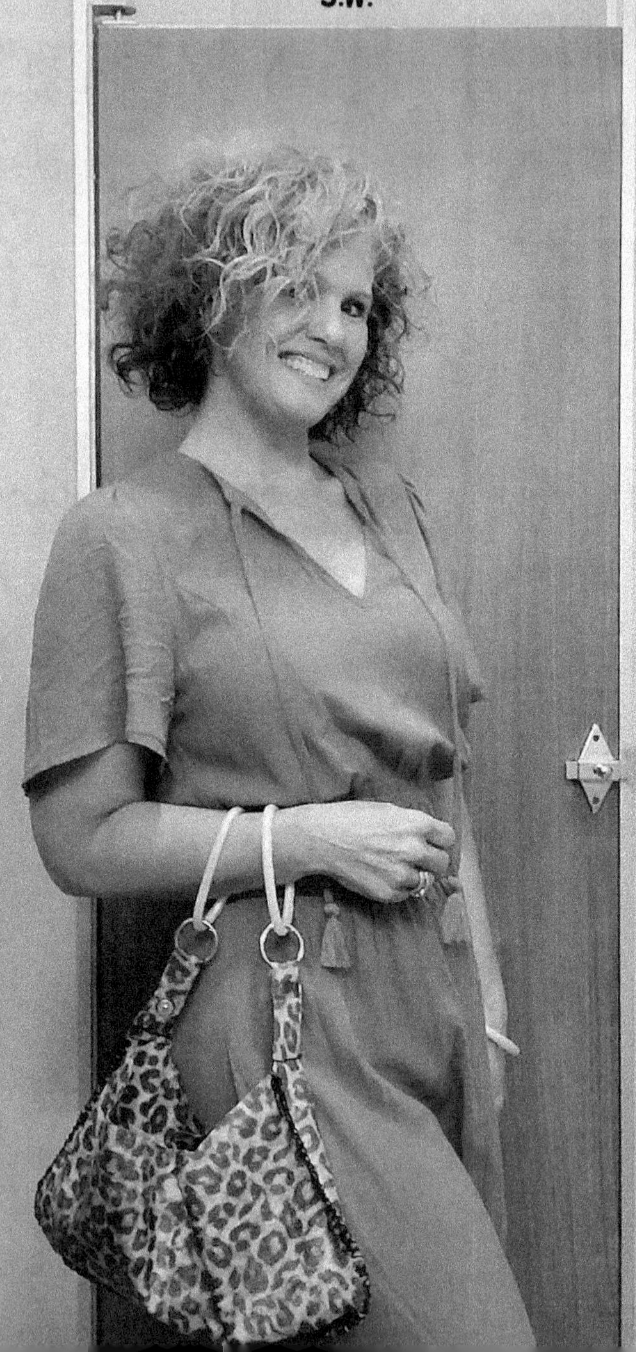
IT DOES NOT HAPPEN OVERNIGHT
BUT ONE DAY IT WILL HAPPEN.
JUST KEEP GOING.

S.W.

The
6 Rules
on
Losing
Weight

Written by

S.W.

Published By
S.W. Creative Designs
and Blurb

Table of Contents

Table of Contents

PREFACE

Have you ever looked in the mirror and said, I wish I could change? I did. I struggled with my weight. I always hid in pictures, never wanting my full body shown. I remember looking in a full length mirror after I had my second child, "I had tree trunks for legs" I told myself. I had many moments of wanting to lose weight. But there was one moment that showed me I was bigger than I thought. After that day I was determined to lose weight. Roller coaster diets and all. Until one day I found my solution. I stop listening to it is "just one bite" voice inside my head. I stopped saying "I will start tomorrow." I kept going and said it will fall off eventually. I just need to stick with it. I am going to wear my skinny jeans with boots that I can zip up past my calves. You have to want it to get it! Yes, it was hard but my end result was worth it. I can wear my skinny jeans and zip up boots. But honestly, nobody is perfect. So do not doubt yourself, when I get that question "how did you do it?" I tell them *full of excitement* my weight loss story. I hope I can help them look in the mirror and not say "they can not do this." I want them to look in the mirror and say "I DID IT!". But remember you are beautiful inside and out, no matter what your final results are. If your happy when you look in the mirror, that is all that matters.

How I felt on my 34th Birthday

It was my birthday I turned 34 and on my way home from work I got pulled over for speeding. As I was waiting I also remembered when I turned 19 and got pulled over. The officer didn't give me a ticket because it was my birthday. So I put on my best smile and rolled down my window. The policeman asked me for my license and registration; I had it ready and gladly gave it to him. *I waited to see his response when he looked at my birthday on my license.* He said, "it's your birthday" and I said "yes it is." He tore off the ticket and gave it to me saying "Happy Birthday and slow down around that curve." I could not believe it, he gave me a ticket on my birthday. Then I looked down and remembered I was 230 pounds verses when I was 19 at 150 pounds. The ticket was because I was speeding and it did not matter if it was my birthday. But in my mind *maybe* it was because I was bigger than I use to be. I felt that was why I did not get out of the ticket on my birthday. When I went home I looked at myself in the mirror naked. My top-half was not as bad as my bottom half. I then focus on my legs, they were the biggest part of my body. I could barely see my knees. I broke down crying. I felt ugly. **I felt ugly on my birthday.** I barely had any clothes that fit me, the clothes that did fit were not the style I wanted. I had a section in my closet I kept, hoping one day I could wear them again.

The diets I tried

I tried many diets. Like many people I tried starving myself. I counted 1000 calories a day. NO FAT...everything I ate was fat free. It worked when I was younger. I told myself "it has got to work again." I still ate skittles and had a diet coke at the movies. I read the package and it hardly had any fat and it was still under the 1000 calories. Months went by and nothing brilliant happened but I did not have the right knowledge of what my body needed. I tried and tried but until I understood my body and have a positive mind set; I would never lose weight and keep it off. I gave up and continue to eat the food my body was use to. Italian food, oh how I loved fried lasagna and bread sticks. The fried lasagna had 1000 calories but I would dip my bread sticks in the fettuccine sauce so I guesstimated that was about 1700 calories. I consumed it and just didn't eat anything else that day. I also had about 5 diet drinks to fill me up when I got hungry again. The other foods my metabolism was use to was southwestern egg rolls and ranch dressing. They only had about 300 calories each but I ate all four not including the ranch. I still counted the calories all the time but again I did not understand what my body and mind needed.

I continued eating the same way for 3 years. I got down to 190 but it fluctuated. The big thing was phentermine to lose weight. It was the talk of the town. I knew 3 people who were taking it and they were losing weight. I finally decided to make a Doctors appointment. This is it! This was going to work, I knew I was overweight at 5'4 weighing 190 LBS. It was my day of the appointment and I was crossing my fingers I would get approved.

This was the first time I wanted to be seen as overweight. I had an ice cream on my way there just in case. I made it to my appointment and waited nervously but excited. *This was going to help me lose weight.* The nurse came out and called my name. I got out of the chair I could barely fit in and walked through the door. The first thing was the weigh in. I didn't even take my shoes off either this time. I weighed in at almost 200. I didn't care even if it was more than I thought this time because I wanted to be fat to get the magic pill. I got all the blood work up done while I was there. *Maybe it was my thyroid,* I thought. I heard an overactive thyroid will make it hard to lose weight. The doctor came in and showed me the chart. I was in the obese section. I was in, I was in the magic pill section! He wrote me a prescription but it had rules to follow with it. 1500 calories a day, no counting fat grams, exercise at least 30 minutes a day, 4 times a week. I still had to count calories and now adding exercise...bummer. But, I had the magic pill! Finally! I took it everyday watching my 1500 calories a day. I didn't change my eating patterns because I had 500 more calories than my starving diet. I also did not exercise like I needed to. I just did sit ups from the 10 minute abs DVD I had. It had been a month of taking the magic pill. I was excited to see the Dr. and see my weight on their scale. I knew I had lost some weight but did not know how much. I was at 180 this time. The doctor asked me my routine and I told him I was counting the 1500 calories a day and doing "exercises." I didn't tell him I would have 2 bags of Cheeto's and it was only ab exercises. I did admit I was still drinking diet drinks. I was addicted to my diet drinks. I was not lying but I needed another months supply. He told me to drink more water. I got my next months supply of phentermine.

Then next month I lost another 10 pounds. I had another appointment and I was still in the overweight section. I got another supply and then the next month I was at 160. I finally got to a number I had not seen in a long time. I was skinner than before I had kids. I pulled out all my old clothes from the closet and they fit! I wanted to put on a fashion show, so I did. But when I went to my last Doctors appointment he didn't give me another prescription, so now I was on my own. Since I did not change my eating habits I started gaining my weight back. Each month I put on weight and I got back up to 230. I gained more weight than I originally started with!

I remember I was at a basketball game watching my oldest daughter play (Once again I had no cute clothes to wear). I had on big sweats and a tee shirt and a guy in the bleachers asked me why I was wearing that. I fumbled for an answer..."I wanted to feel comfortable." I started calling my sweats my comfy pants. I even made up a dance for my kids. Singing to them saying "my comfy pants, my comfy pants". I started another starving diet. This time I started walking.

I love my sunrises and sunsets. So I decided to walk around them. I also started listening to people around me talking about different ways to lose weight. I started to change my eating habits. The starving diet apparently was not working. My friend kept telling me diet drinks were bad for me. I did not believe it. *Why would diet drinks be bad?* Diet drinks had no calories and not fat. It helped fill me up when I was hungry. I kept drinking the diet drinks but started eating more good fat and less sugar. The sugar was the hardest to give up. I LOVED my skittles. But this time I changed my skittles to nuts. I had a variety of flavors so I wouldn't eat sugar.

Cashews, pistachios, almonds, walnuts. I would have carb free yogurt instead of regular. I started using sweet drops replacing Aspartame and sugar.

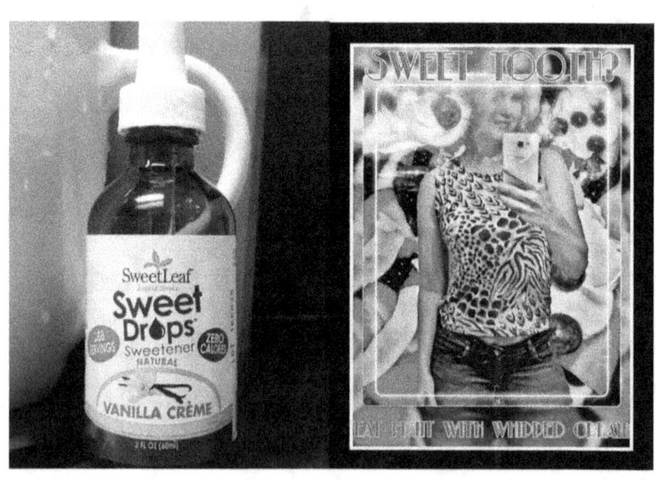

The 6 Rules on Losing Weight
RULE#1

1. **It is not a diet.** It is changing the way you eat. If you can eat fast food every day then you can change.

2. It is not all about working out.

3. You need fat to be skinny.

4. Replace sugar with something better.

5. Quit Diet Cokes because first rule; this is not a diet.

6. Glamour Shots.

I am not a Doctor or specialist and this is not a diet. This is my story on how I lost 100 pounds and kept it off without surgery. People asked me "how I did it?" and this is how I did it.

If you "think" you are on a diet then you will not accomplish your desired weight loss. Diets, in my opinion, are temporary. After you lose the weight fast then you feel like you can eat the way you use to. You will gain the weight back because you have not changed your metabolic system. Your body works like a machine; everything has something it needs. If it does not need it, it will store it, thinking you will need it later. That is why you need to change your system. Everyones system is different. When you find out how it works then you can oil the parts that are needed and feed it so it will burn faster. It won't store it.

Working out helps you achieve staying strong but what you eat feeds your body. Walking is a great way to relieve stress and keep your parts oiled. Find a time that you can spend on yourself walking and enjoy life. It does not have to be 5 hours a day. You just need 30 minutes. Routine is the key. Get yourself in a routine. At first you can chart out your own meals through for day.

Then once you get in your routine it will be a part of life.

Instead of eating a candy bar replace it with something that is lower in sugar. There are so many things out there that's better for you. Cashews, pistachios, lower sugar yogurt, low sugar protein bars, low sugar pies you can make yourself. *(Cashews are a natural way to help anxiety).*

Instead of a soda drink carbonated water. If you like them sweet then add sweet drops. For caffeine you can have coffee with heavy whipping cream and sweet drops.

If you eat fast food make them change it to your meal. Example: Nacho Salad at Taco Bueno; Have them separate the chips and cheese from the meal. Then you can add what is needed. You are in control.

<u>Rule#1.</u>
It is not a diet. It is changing the way you eat. If you can eat fast food every day then you can change.

Did you know?

Did you know that your body is made to break down 30 to 60 grams of sugar a day. Everything after that is stored. SO if you drink just one soda, you are pretty much going to store the rest of the sugar you take in that day. *Unless you go work out like a beast for hours.* But just think if you change your system then your body will be a burning machine. You can go to the gym and just have fun working out. You just need 20 to 30 minutes of fun and you do not have to go every day.

It took me 4 years to figure out what works for me. I did not give up. Finally one day it started falling off. Each month I lost a few pounds but the inches where showing me my results. I can only tell you the feeling I had was **"It is working"** and it pushed me to keep going. The trigger that helped me drop my first 10 pounds was, **I STOPPED DRINKING DIET COKES**! I was not on a diet, I was changing my system. I **believe** the diet cokes were tricking my system into thinking I needed to store sugar even if it was sugar free. I started changing my sweet tooth to a hand full of cashews. Cashews are also high in *GOOD* fat so your body will love you for it. Then if I needed something sweet I would eat a low sugar protein bar or (at first) my favorite was the Atkins Coconut bars. But you need to make sure you can tolerate sugar alcohol. It can make you feel sick if you over eat. Now my favorite bar is the Power Crunch. It has no sugar alcohol and it is low in sugar. It helps me get passed the sugar addiction when I craved it.

Now I hear this a lot "I don't drink diet cokes or eat sugar." That is when you need to put the Fitness Pal on your phone. You need to chart everything you put into your body. You will be amazed at how many foods have an over abundance of sugar. Then you can change it or replace it by making better choices. Once you figure out what your system does not need, you will be saying "IT IS WORKING!" and you will push yourself to keep going with out surgery and diet pills

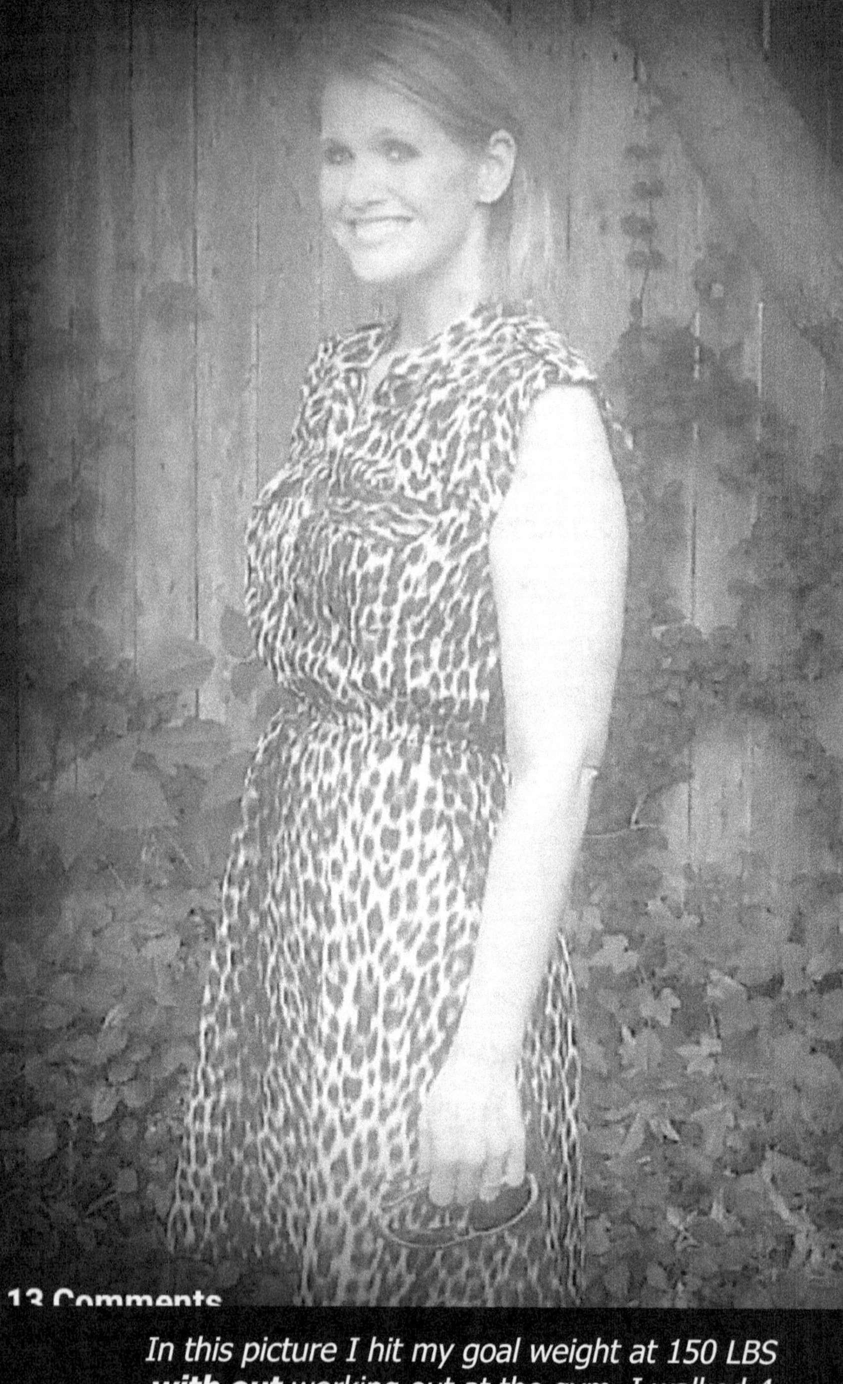

13 Comments
In this picture I hit my goal weight at 150 LBS
with out working out at the gym. I walked 4
times a week for 30 to 45 minutes.

It Does make a difference

What you eat will make a difference. I see it time and time again.

THAT ONE PIECE OF CANDY

THAT ONE PIECE OF CAKE

"Is it worth all your hard work changing the way you eat to go back to the old way?"

It does matter if you eat that. Because you get off your routine. Now it is OK to try it, a small bite but don't eat the whole piece. My psychology is *if you have eaten it before THEN you KNOW it taste good but it is not what your body needs.*

I mean come on...SUGAR is good but if you can make a cake and CHANGE out the sugar to a sugar substitute why would you not do that. *Isn't it what you want?* Diabetics have to do it to stay healthy. If you want to change your body, you have to change the way you feed it.

That was Then and this is Now

This is what I would tell people when they asked...HOW DID YOU DO IT?

Then

I used to drink 4 diet cokes a day, so I stopped that. I used to eat 20 fat grams with 1000 calories, now I eat 60 to 80 fat grams with 1500 to 1800 calories. But the calories are not the goal. I stopped eating my favorite candy and eating nuts in their place. So basically I eat 60 to 80 fat grams, I don't count my calories and 60 to 160 carbs a day. No more bread. I use to eat sandwiches everyday...it was low in calories but high in carbs. Then I started walking 30 to 45 minutes 2 to 4 times a week. You can download the fitness pal to monitor the fat, carbs, protein and sugars. I feel like before my body would hold onto the fat when I didn't eat enough. Now my body thinks I have enough and I think my metabolism is working better. I tried so many diets, diet pills and I think the over the counter pills confuses my metabolism.

Now

NO CANDY, NO DIET COKES or FRIES.

That is an ice breaker for me. I simply kept my routine. I tell people it is not a diet; it's a way of life. You have to be willing to change what society has set in your mind. Countless commercials of food that looks delicious but so unhealthy for you. You can eat delicious food but you have to change the ingredient's. I make a really heavenly low carb coconut cream pie. You can have a lot of amazing food you just have to tweak it. Like I said before ***it is not a diet it is a way of changing your system***. If you do not want to change then just put this book down. Put yourself back on a diet. In my opinion, it won't work because diets are a trick just like diet cokes. You think your are doing good because you are drinking a diet coke but your not. Your wasting your time on being on a diet. It won't last. You will gain back what you lost plus some when you go back to eating the old way. ***Eating the way that made you want to go on a diet.*** If you change you will never have to go on a diet again!!!!!! How nice that would be...

My Routine meal plan

Morning

2 Scrambled Eggs and Bacon Well Done

Or Protein Smoothie

You can still eat fast food you just need to change it up. When you do go to McDonald's you order a side of eggs and a side of bacon.

You can make your own protein drink. You buy a good protein powder, your favorite frozen fruit, Greek or carb master yogurt and unsweetened almond or coconut milk

1 cup Frozen Fruit

1 cup Unsweetened Almond or Coconut Milk

3 Tablespoons of Yogurt

1 Scoop Protein Powder or follow the directions on the label.

Blend away in your blender until it is nice and smooth.

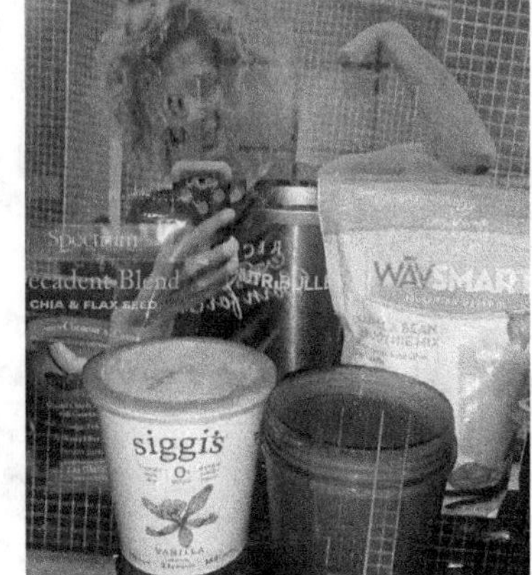

Snack

A handful of Cashews (or any variety of nuts), protein bar or Carb master Yogurt

*My Variety of Nuts: Cashews, Pistachios, Peanuts, Almonds, Walnuts and Pecans.

My Protein Bars: Adkins Coconut Bar, Power Crunch, Kind Bars (that say 5 sugars) and Quest Bars.

They have so many different protein bars out there you just need to read the label to make sure it is not high in sugar. Good Carbs are OK.

My Yogurt: Carbmaster Vanilla Yogurt from Kroger or the Zero Vanilla Greek Yogurt.

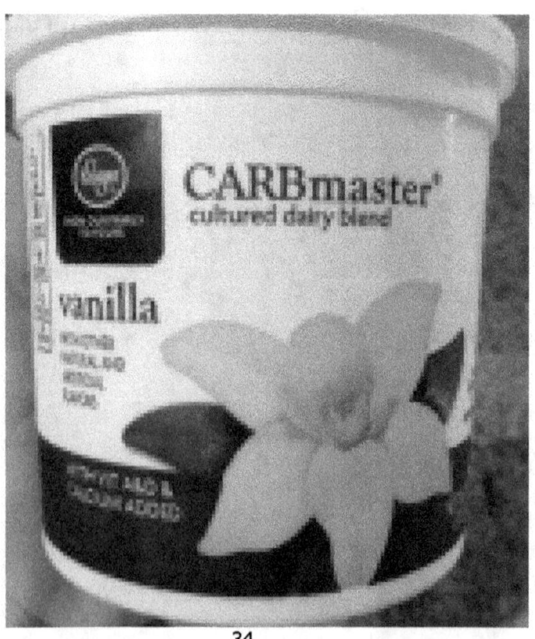

Lunch

Chick-Fil-A Cobb Salad with Grilled Nuggets and Ranch dressing.

It is easy to eat healthy when you are on the go. When you go to a fast food or restaurant always change it to what you need to eat healthy.

Example: Taco Bueno Nacho Salad

"Can I please have a Nacho Salad with the chips and queso on the side. I would also like an extra side of taco meat. I would also like jalapeños and hot sauce please."

If you order it that way, you can add a few chips and a little queso on top. You have control of your Nacho Salad.

Then check your bag because sometimes they do get confused. You are paying for it out of your pocket and if it is wrong you will pay for it later in your stomach.

Afternoon Snack

A hand full of Cashews, protein bar or Carbmaster Yogurt.

Dinner

Turkey Roll Ups, Tuna Salad Sandwich, Nacho Salad or Salad with Grilled Chicken and Salad Dressing

***My Salad Dressing:** Ranch, it is my favorite because it is low in sugar and it gives me my fat. You can use any dressing you like as long as the sugar is low.

It is the weekend plan:

You can go to any restaurant and find something that is healthy and good to eat. Sometimes take your own food in to take the place of something they don't have.

Example: You go to Chuy's and you want to eat Flour tortilla's with queso. Bring your own Low Carb Flour tortilla's. Pull them suckers right out of your purse and dip it in the delicious queso or the famous jalapeño ranch they serve. Get the chicken or beef fajitas and use the Low Carb Flour Tortilla's. When you do change your system to burn what you don't need then you can have chips and hot sauce too but take out a portion of the chips to make sure you do not over eat them. Use your Fitness pal app to see how many. My portion is about 15 chips for me.

Example: You go to a birthday party. Scan the table for the food you can eat. Turkey, if it is in a sandwich, take off the bread. Nuts, carrots, pickles, ranch, fruit, cheese there are lots of things you can eat. Then the cake comes out...I do not get a piece because I think to myself **how many pieces of cake have I eaten in my life and is it worth it?** I say no thank you and pull out my protein bar. It takes the place of the sweet for me. I do not leave the party thinking *why did I eat that piece of cake.* Now people like to drink socially. Well you can drink but I do not drink over two beers. I do not drink the fruity drinks because it has too much sugar. Heineken is a lower carb beer and no sugar. Now you can use your fitness pal or Google what is lower in carbs. ONCE YOU GET YOUR ROUTINE DOWN you do not have to Google nutrients or rely on your app.

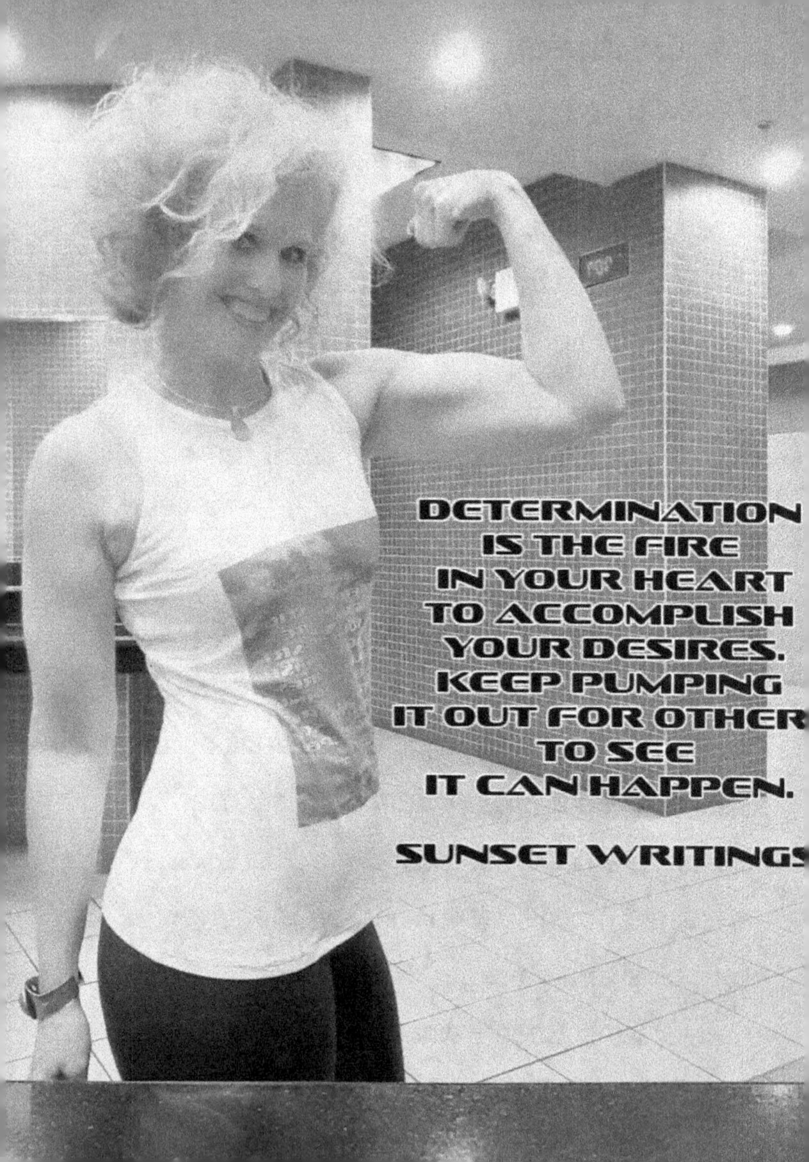

DETERMINATION
IS THE FIRE
IN YOUR HEART
TO ACCOMPLISH
YOUR DESIRES.
KEEP PUMPING
IT OUT FOR OTHER
TO SEE
IT CAN HAPPEN.

SUNSET WRITINGS

It Takes Time
RULE#2

It takes time for your body to switch geers. Everyone is different but you will know it when it happens. If you do not follow the coarse and you eat a piece of candy or piece of cake then you pretty much have to start over. The whole goal is to change your system so later you can have a little more every now and then but your body will burn it off instead of storing it.

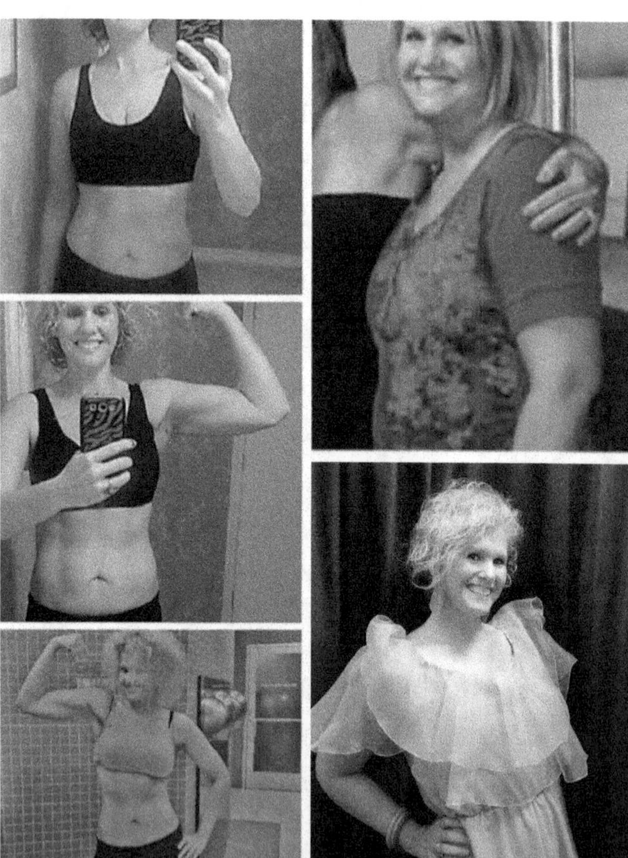

Now don't give up on what you just read because after you change your system through time you can add more to your daily routine. Remember if you can eat the same fast food every day you can change your routine and then when you get bored "change it up." Once you figure out your wall that kept you from loosing the weight your body will not store the sugar and fat.

Example: I can eat popcorn and drink a coke zero at the movies! I couldn't do that in the beginning because I was changing my metabolic rate.

Now when "I decide" to eat something my body is not use to it will burn it faster than before because I was stuck behind that wall. I had to bust through by not giving up so it would work! You can not go back to old habits and over indulge because then you have to start over. Stop telling yourself "I am on a diet." You have to have the right mind set to accomplish your goal. You are changing your fuel system. Keep reading and find out some of my data I kept while using fitness pal. I only looked at the protein, carbs, fat and sugar. I did not count the calories. It helped me regulate my fuel for the day. **My burning fuel.**

<u>Rule#2.</u>
It is not all about working out.

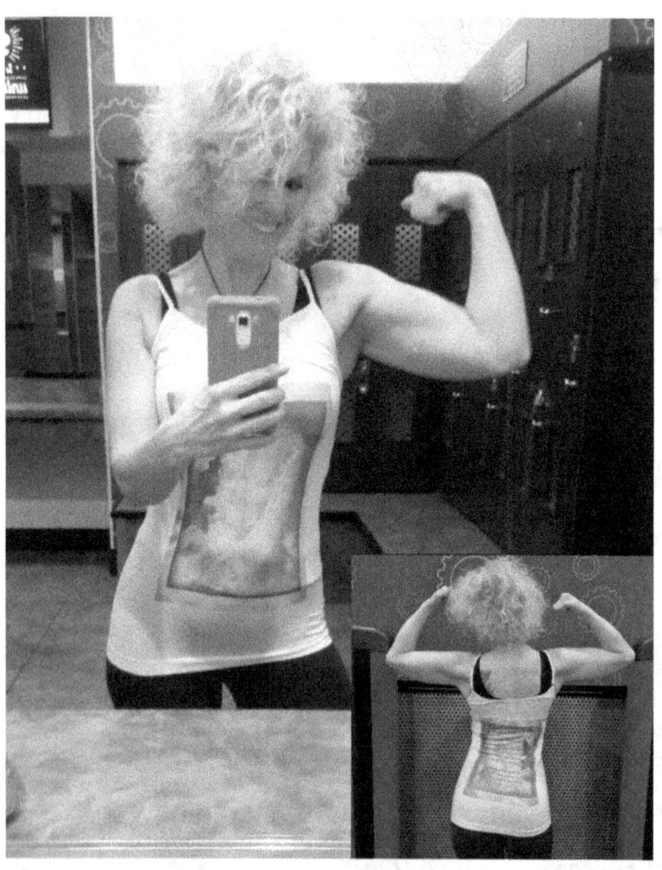

My Fitness Pal
RULE#3

October 20, 2011

My first fitness pal input started in October 2011. I saw I could do it. I just needed to figure out how to balance my system. I liked everything but needed more fat and protein.

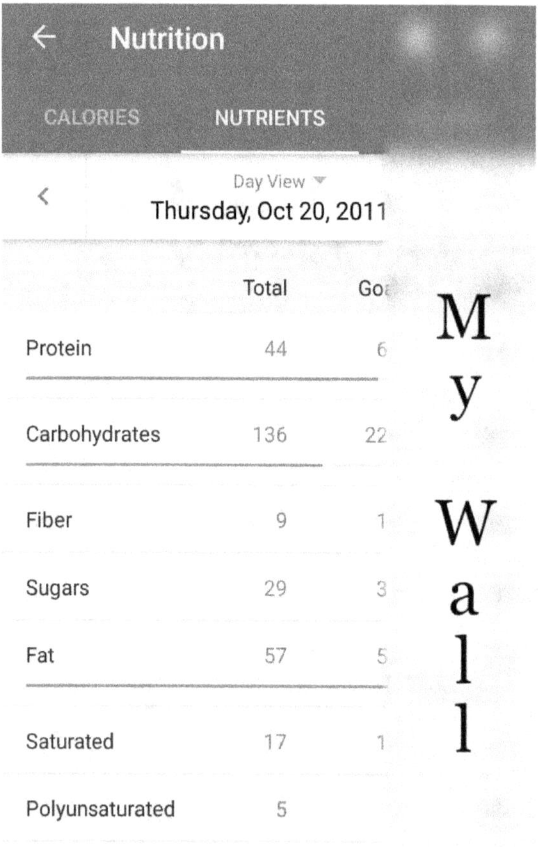

Nutrition

CALORIES   NUTRIENTS

Day View ▼
Thursday, Oct 20, 2011

	Total	Goal
Protein	44	6
Carbohydrates	136	22
Fiber	9	1
Sugars	29	3
Fat	57	5
Saturated	17	1
Polyunsaturated	5	

My Wall

November 1, 2011

This was a bad input because my sugar was way too high and I needed a lot more fat. That is when it occurred to me what my body intake was. What my spike was. I had started loosing weight. My calculated balance is what I went off of.

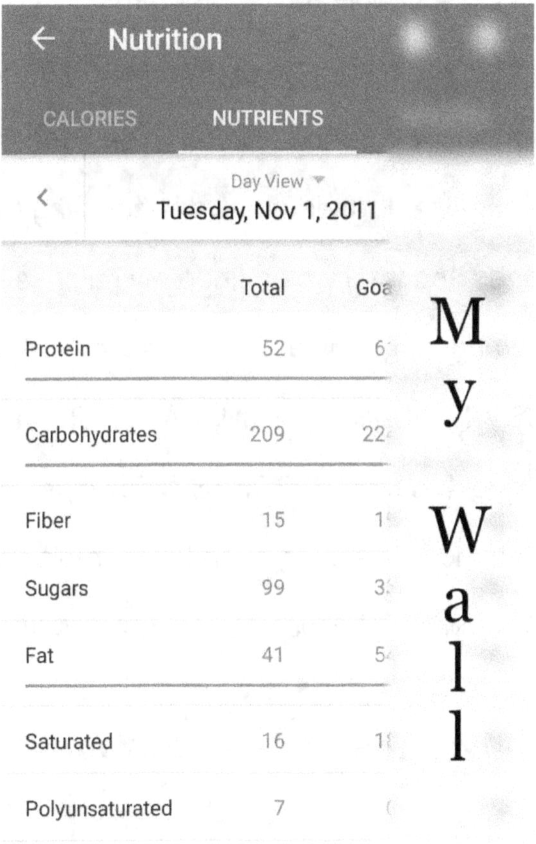

Nutrition		
CALORIES	NUTRIENTS	
Day View		
Tuesday, Nov 1, 2011		
	Total	Goal
Protein	52	6
Carbohydrates	209	22
Fiber	15	1
Sugars	99	3
Fat	41	5
Saturated	16	1
Polyunsaturated	7	

I realized what my wall was. Sugar, I loved sugar. *My wall was...it is low in fat and calories.* I said to myself "If I watch my calories and fat I am maintaining my diet." But my calories were not the real problem, it was the sugar. My sugar was off the chart. Did you know most people have 300 grams of sugar a day? I read your body is only made to break down 30 to 60 grams of sugar a day depending on your size. I would go all day counting my calories and fat. I would keep my calories at 1200 and fat grams at 20 grams a day. WHICH WAS WHY WAS I GAINING WEIGHT. Then drinking 4 to 6 DIET COKES a day made my system go into storing everything I ate because HOLY SMOKES, I was **starving my**self!!!!

<u>Rule#3</u>
You need fat to be skinny!!

November 8, 2011

My Wall just needed a protein bar or protein drink to have it perfect.

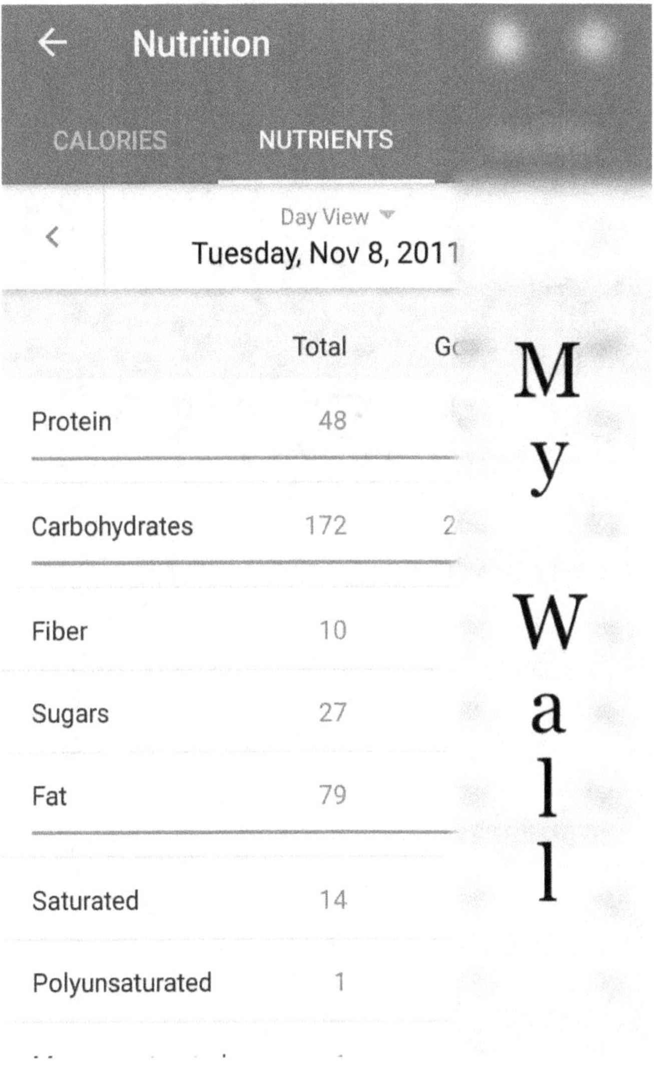

	Total	Goal
Protein	48	
Carbohydrates	172	2
Fiber	10	
Sugars	27	
Fat	79	
Saturated	14	
Polyunsaturated	1	

My Wall

My Perfect Fuel Chart
RULE#4

Sept 2018

For breakfast I went to Denny's with my best friend. I had half of an ultimate omelette, 3 tablespoons of grits mixed with butter and salt (I mix my eggs with grits), half an english muffin, 2 servings of black coffee with splenda and 4 french vanilla creamer cups.

	Total
Protein	75
Carbohydrates	103
Fiber	11
Sugars	33
Fat	99
Saturated	24
Polyunsaturated	2

My Wall

Breakfast at Denny's

1/2 Ultimate Omelette
Sugar 1 Grams
Carbs 2.5 Grams
Fat 28 Grams
Protein 18 Grams

Grits
Sugar 0 Gram
Carbs 11 Grams
Fat 0.7 Grams
Protein 1.2 Grams

Coffee and Splenda
Zero Sugar
*(*my preferred sugar substitute is Stevia or sweet drops)*

French Vanilla Creamer
Sugar 20 Grams
Carbs 20 Grams
Fat 6 Grams
Protein 0 Gram
*(*my preferred creamer is heavy whipping cream or sugar free French Vanilla Creamer)*

1/2 English Muffin
Sugar 0.5 Grams
Carbs 12.5 Grams
Fat 0.5 Grams
Protein 2 Grams

<u>## Snacks on the go</u>

Nature Valleys Peanut Butter Protein Bar

Sugar 6 Grams
Carbs 14 Grams
Fat 12 Grams
Protein 10 Grams

No lunch because I had a big breakfast and early dinner

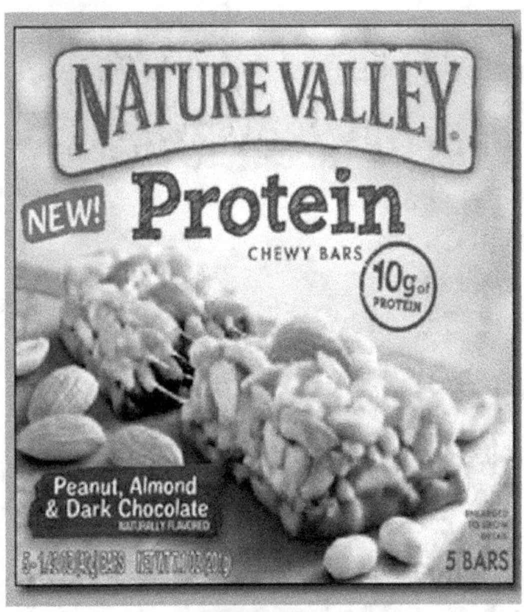

<u>*Rule#4.*</u>
Replace sugar with something better

Dinner at Razzoo's

For dinner I went to Razzoo's with my kids. It was an early dinner around 4:30.
Fried Pickles, Chopped Salad with Blacken Chicken and Ranch with Water.

Chopped Salad with Blacken Chicken

Sugar 2 Grams
Carbs 11 Grams
Fat 34 Grams
Protein 32 Grams

Fried Pickles (about 10 pickles)

Sugar 2.4 Grams
Carbs 30 Grams
Fat 3.6 Grams
Protein 5.5 Grams

Ranch 4 TBSP

Sugar 1 Gram
Carbs 2 Grams
Fat 14 Grams

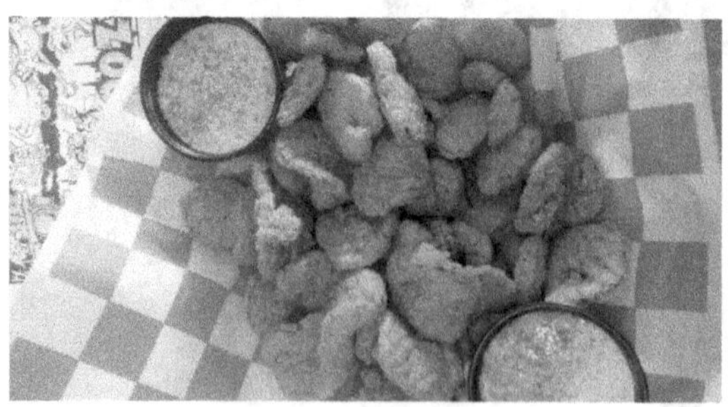

Quick Recipes

Low Carb Pepperoni Hot Pocket

If you want a Hot Pocket Pizza but not the carbs and sugar this is just as easy to make. It is kind of like a homemade hot pocket but not as bad.

2 carb balance tortilla, 8 pepperoni slices, 1/4 cup Italian blend cheese. Then use a George Forman or heat it up on the stove to cook it and it will be crispy.

270 calories

17 fat

6 carbs

1 sugars

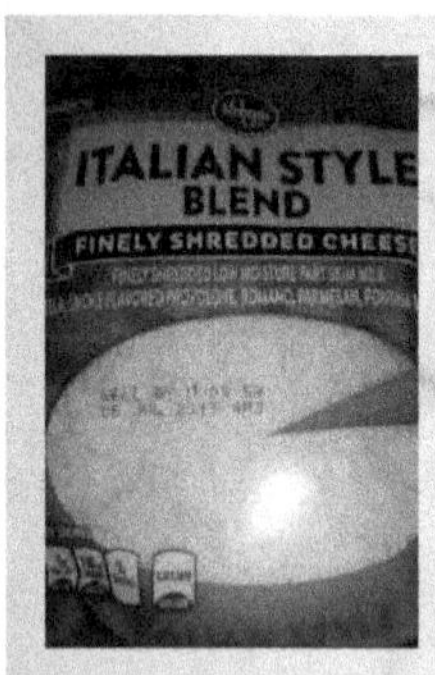

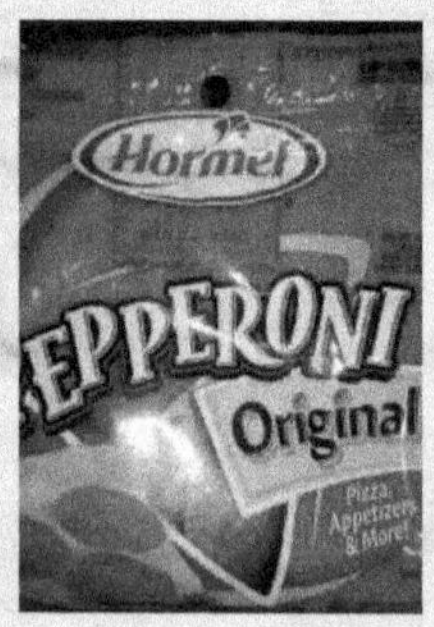

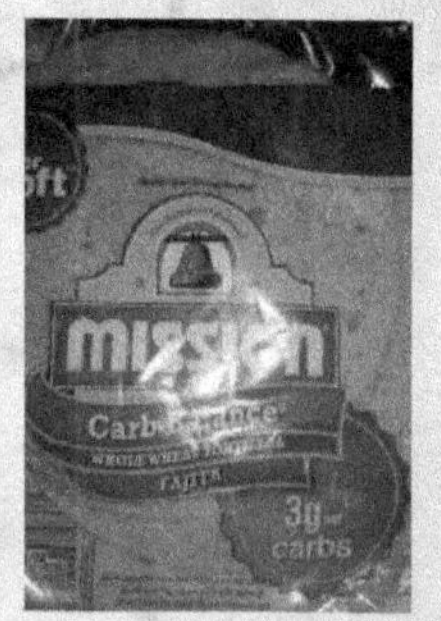

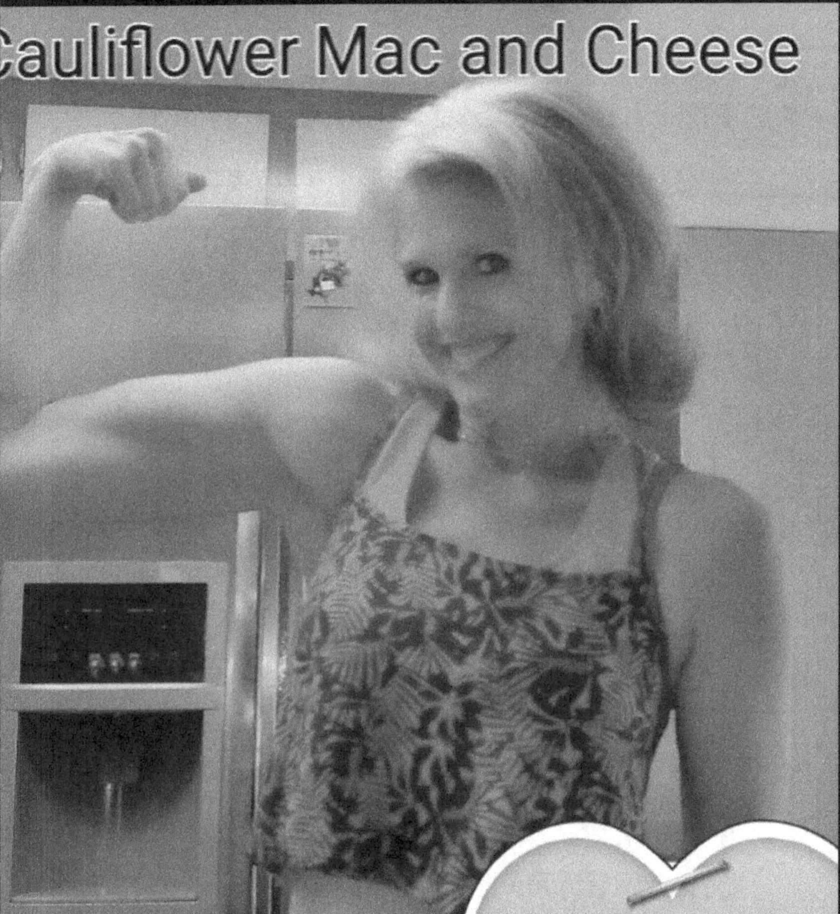

Cauliflower Mac and Cheese
Strength is in your hands
but
Willpower is in your mind
Sunset Writings

Cauliflower Mac and Cheese

Take one head of cauliflower and break into small pieces. Rinse off well. Boil a pot of water. Place the small pieces of cauliflower in boiling water until they are tender. Drain water. Turn warmer on low. Add whipping cream, yogurt butter (or cream cheese), cheese, salt and pepper. Mix well. Let cook for about 5 minutes and it is Ready. Then if you want you can add cheese on top and bake in the oven to melt cheese. Like a casserole. Also you can add bacon for more protein.

1 Head of Cauliflower
1 Cup of Heavy Whipping Cream
2 Oz of Cream Cheese OR 1 tbsp of Yogurt Butter
1 1/2 Cup of Shredded Cheddar Cheese
(use can use any kind of cheese as long as it shredded)
Salt and Pepper
Bacon optional

Low Sugar Key Lime Pie

Pie crust: Take 1 cup of unsalted raw sunflower seeds and grind them into flour consistency. Then add 1 cup of Swerve sugar substitute, 1 cup of soften butter and 2 cups of unsweetened shredded coconut. Grind all ingredients together. Next lightly grease your dish or pan. Add crust mixture and pat down evenly with a fork. Second you make the pie filling.

Filling: Take 2 large ripe avocados, remove the pit and scoop out the inside, 4 oz of cream cheese and blend together with mixer until smooth. Add 1 and a half cups of Swerve or Sugar Substitute, half a cup of sour cream, 1 cup of heavy whipping cream then squeeze 4 limes for juice into mixture, (taste test to see if you need more tart/lime Juice.) Mix all the ingredients together. Finally, you place filling into pie crust. Add cool whip if desired. Place in refrigerator to chill for 2 to 3 hours.

Crust

1 Cup Unsalted Raw Sunflower Seeds

1 Cup of soften Butter

2 Cups of Unsweetened Shredded Coconut

1 Cup of Swerve or Sugar Substitute

Filling

4 oz Cream Cheese

2 Large Ripe Avocados

4 Limes

1/2 Cup Sour Cream

1 Cup of Heavy Whipping Cream

1.5 Cups of Swerve or Sugar Substitute

Topping
Cool Whip (optional)

Low Carb Chocolate Cream Pie

Place heavy whipping cream, coconut milk and eggs yolks into a sauce pan and heat up to mixture. Mix well. Take your blended or finely chopped unsweetened baking chocolate, xylitol, Stevia and add in mixture. Stir until chocolate is melted. Then slowly add in xanthan gum while constantly whisking over low heat. (it will get clumpy if you don't blend slow) Bring to a boil and let mixture boil for a minute. Remove form heat. Stir in the butter and vanilla. You can make homemade cream with 2 cups of heavy whipping cream and half a cup of sugar substitute or buy cool whip. For the crust I use a low carb crust.

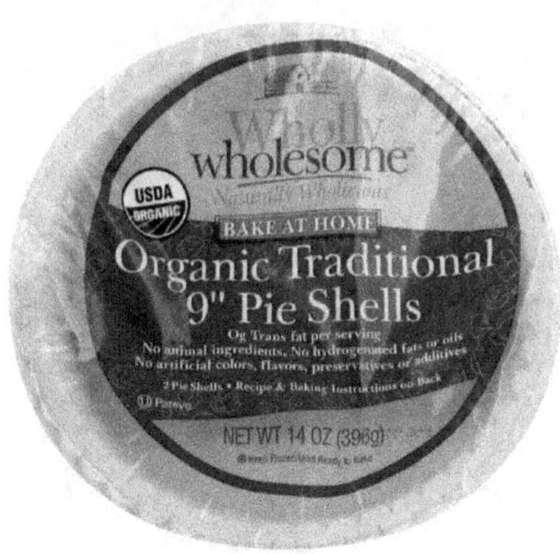

Pie Filling

1 cup heavy whipping cream

1 cup teaspoon of coconut milk

3/4 cup powdered xylitol

1 1/2 xantham gum

2 oz unsweetened baking chocolate

chopped finely

Cool Whip for topping or homemade whip

cream (2 cups of heavy whipping cream and

half a cup of sugar substitute. Mix with mixer

until peaks form and thickness.)

Crust

1 low carb pre-made crust and follow

directions.

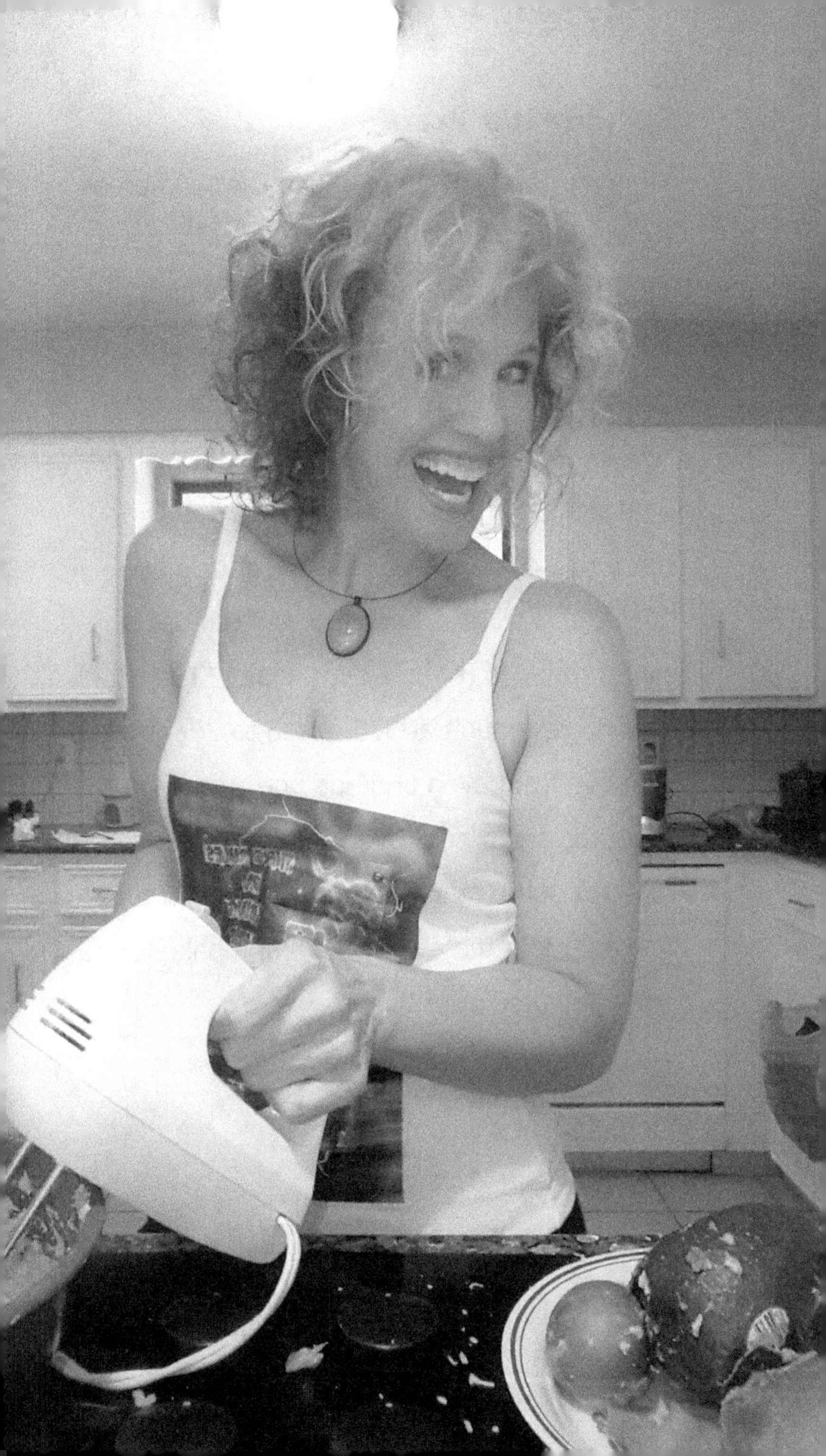

Cauliflower Pizza

First you take a head of cauliflower and break it into florets. Rinse and Dry. Place dry florets into the microwave for 6 minutes or until soft. Let cool. Then blend into rice size. Next squeeze any extra juice out. In a large bowl mix together the beaten eggs, cheeses and seasonings. Then take cauliflower dough and pat into a circle on a cookie sheet or pizza stone. You will still have moisture so use a paper towel to remove extra water. Then cook cauliflower dough at 375 for 15 to 20 minutes. Remove from oven and add your toppings. My favorites are, black olives, sun dried tomatoes, and spinach. Then add more cheese on top. Place back in the oven at 375 and bake for 10 to 15 minutes or until done.

Cauliflower crust

One head of cauliflower

1 beaten egg

1 cup of grated mozzarella cheese

1/4 cup of grated Parmesan cheese

1/2 tsp garlic salt or dried garlic (optional)

Toppings (optional)

Blacks Olives

Sun-dried Tomatoes

Spinach

Pepperoni

More cheese

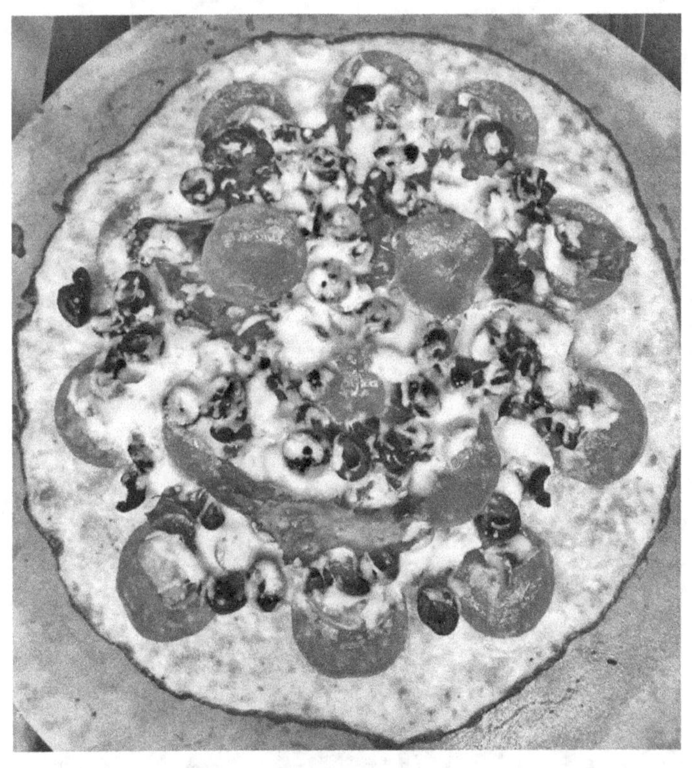

Those are just some of the things I love to make and feel good about. But there are many healthy ways to eat good things. Plus they are so easy to make. I am going off topic. THIS IS NOT A DIET YOU ARE CHANGING THE WAY YOU EAT!

But there are a lot of things to help your sweet tooth and keep your body burning fat.

Here are more of my favorites; low sugar coconut cream pie, low sugar pecan pie, low sugar chocolate cupcakes. These all helped my sweet tooth and I could take it to the birthday party and everyone will love you for it.

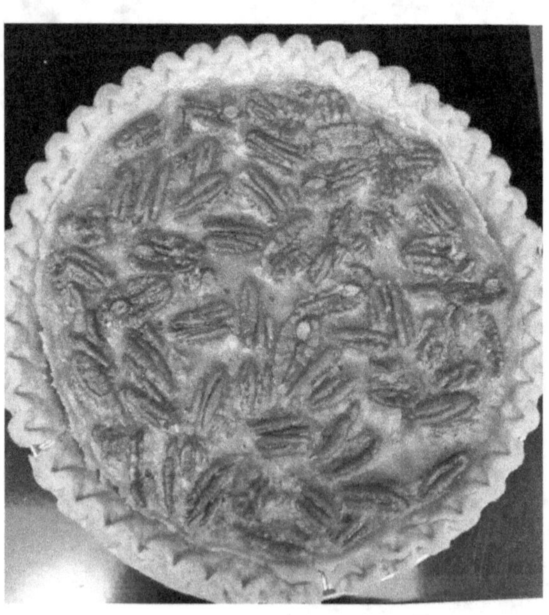

This is a before and after picture of me changing my system. This is an actually post from my FB January 14, 2018. It really makes you feel good when you see the difference. THAT IS WHY YOU TAKE BEFORE AND AFTER PICTURES! If you don't see it in the mirror you can see yourself change in pictures. When you lose weight you want to show yourself and others your hard work and what determination means. It means ACCOMPLISHMENT! I am eating my low sugar pecan pie in this picture.

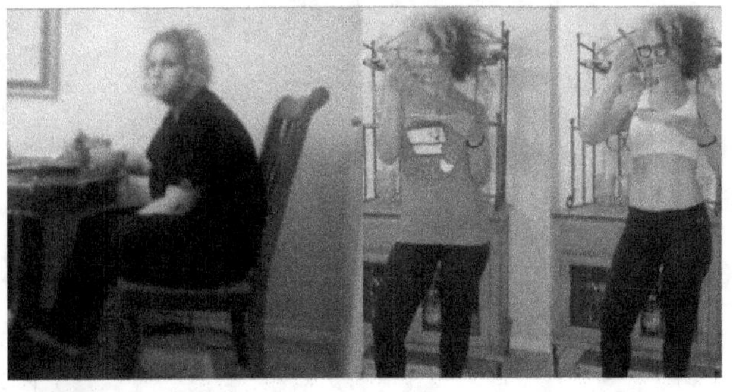

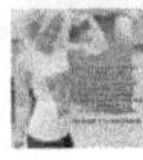

When you never used to like to take photos of yourself because of you and then someone made you feel good about it. I was going through my sunset pictures and found these. Nothing is impossible, just have to find out what works for you. It is not easy on what you invision but with hard work and discipline it just might happen. This is with anything you desire in your heart.

Quick Tips

Quick tips on how to change

*Body Armour LITE instead of Juice

*Carbonated water and bring your low sugar flavoring to add instead of Soda.

*Want to eat flour tortillas take your own low carb to restaurants.

*Always have your favorite low sugar/carb snack at hand for emergency sweet tooth or hunger.

*If you are not sure about a meal, ask for everything on the side. Then you can add amount of what you want at restaurants or fast food drive thrus. Be in control.

*Almond or Coconut Milk instead Milk.

*Sweet Drops (my favorite), Stevia or Splenda for sweetener.

*Drink water daily.

*Braum's Sugar free bread instead of regular bread.

*Twisted Spiral Sweet Potato or Squash instead of Pasta.

Quick Fast Food Choices for Lunch and Dinner

Taco Bueno
Nacho Salad with Chips and Queso on the side.
Extra side of Taco Meat

or 2 or 3 Taco but everything separated throw the shell away and use your carb master tortillas instead of their shell or flour.

Chick Fil A
Cobb Salad with Grilled Chicken Nuggets and Ranch Dressing.

Chicken Noodle Soup and Salad with Ranch (add 4 piece grilled nuggets to salad if desired).

Jack in the Box
They serve breakfast all day.

Side of Scrambled eggs and 2 Sides of Bacon crumble the bacon in the eggs and ask for picante sauce if desired or the Chicken Fajitas Pita is OK every now and then.

Braums
Single or double meat, cheese, pickles, extra pickles and bacon with no bun (add mustard and a little ketchup if desired).

Panda Express

Small or Medium Mushroom Chicken a la carte with one egg roll and soy sauce. (NO RICE) If you want the meal add vegetable mix.

Sonic

Foot long Coney with chili and cheese NO BUN or Hamburger with NO BUN (but there bun less hamburgers come in weird container, harder to eat out of). They also have really good carbonated water and you can add one of their sugar free flavors.

Wendy's

Hamburger with NO BUN or Southwestern Avocado Salad with regular Ranch, Taco Salad and ONLY USE 4 CHIPS, crumble them up if desired. Throw the rest away so you won't be tempted.

*At Restaurants use the same philosophy. Grocery Store's ALWAYS READ THE LABELS on new things you want to try. It might say it is low sugar or healthy but sometimes it is not. Now I talked about some things you can make but sometimes you don't want to make everything. You can get things already pre made. They have cauliflower mash potatoes, Broccoli cheese and cauliflower rice, lots of things to choose from. You just need to be smarter than the label and read it.

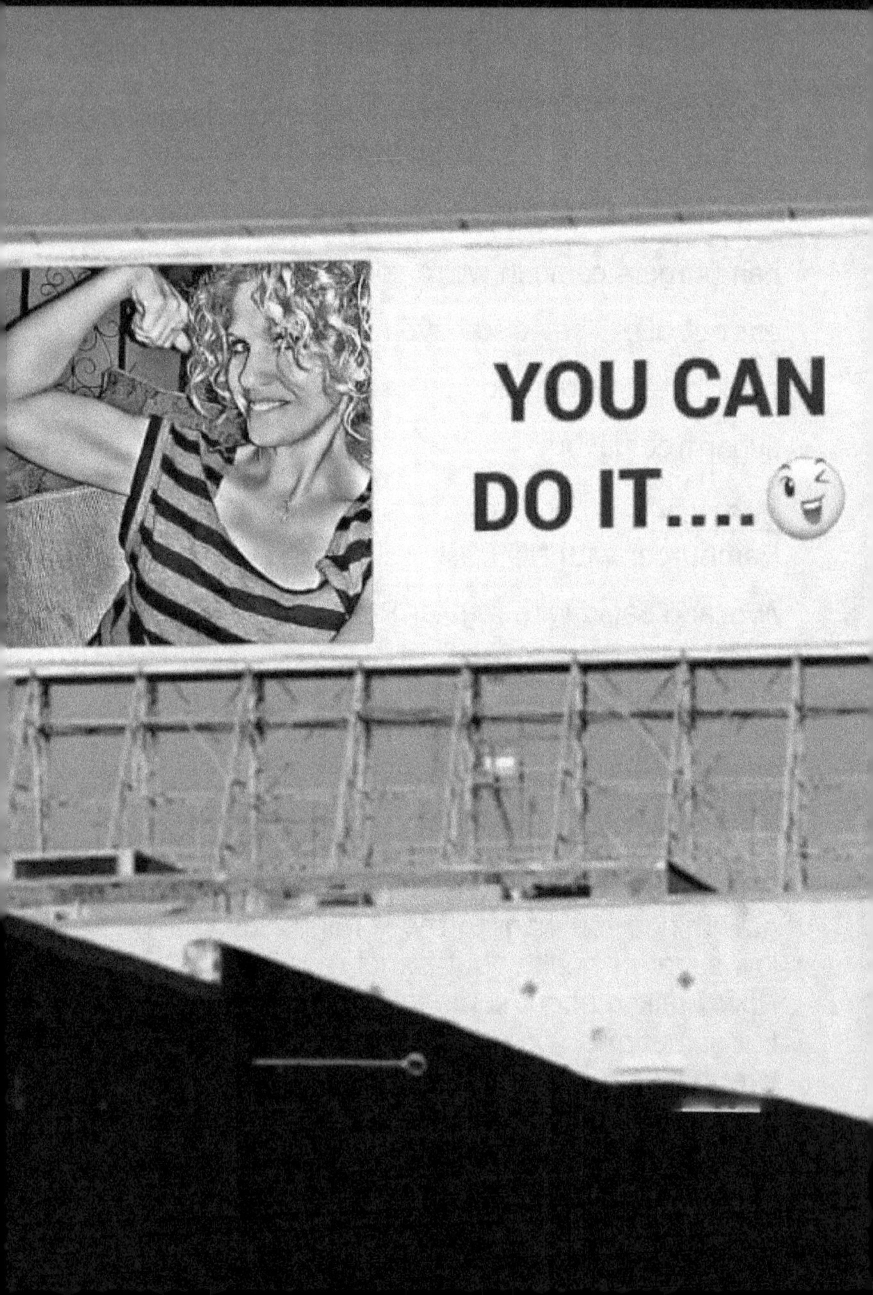

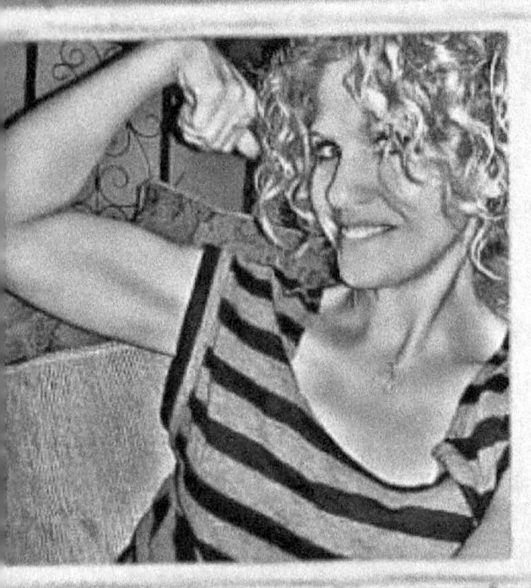

YOU CAN
DO IT.....

Yes You Can

*You can eat a hamburger just ask for bun-less

*You can eat a breakfast burrito just ask for no tortilla and put it in your low carb tortilla

*You can eat Chinese food just get mushroom chicken, string bean, cashew chicken with no rice. Add an egg roll with soy sauce if desired.

*You can eat a foot long with chili and cheese just ask for no bun

*You can eat tacos from your favorite mexican place but use your carb master tortillas instead of their shell or flour

Snap Kitchen

Snap Kitchen is my favorite healthy place to eat lunch on the go. They have a lot different varieties of meals and snacks to choose from. Below is a list of my favorite fuel choices.

Breakfast
Cheesy Egg Bites
Turkey Chili Scramble
AB and J Oatmeal

Lunch or Dinner
Cranberry Pecan Chicken Salad Wrap
Garlic Roasted Cauliflower
Crispy Chicken
Naked Chicken
Chicken Chili Enchiladas
Over Easy Burger with Sweet Potato Wedges
Turkey Chili with Cheese

They have lots of different meals and snacks to try when you are changing your fuel system.

My Moment that kept me going

Many of my diets and attempts to lose weight were zumba, diet pills, starving myself and Atkins. I didn't see long lasting results. With Zumba, maybe I lost a few pounds. With Diet Pills, I did lose 40 pounds but I gained back 70. Starving myself was the hardest because I did not see the results time after time pulling my hair saying **"why is this not working!"** I got frustrated after I tried Atkins. Now, I am not a big meat person so I hated it. Plus I was still drinking my diet cokes. On all these diets and attempts I was still drinking the diet cokes.

Then I started walking. I got up to walking for 45 minutes 4 to 5 times a week. It was something that was fun. Outside was my freedom. I did not lose any weight but it did not matter as much because I like to be outside. Looking at unique, beautiful things and taking photos. Then I quit the diet cokes and started watching my sugar. Then one month after walking for several months I noticed something. I was **losing weight**. I decided step on the scale and see. There it was, 10 pounds down. Maybe my friend was

right? The diet cokes are bad for me. Then
after I paid attention and found out what my
wall was, my fat started to fall off. Every
month I would lose pounds. It was only a few
pounds but I was still losing inches. People
started to notice.

**_I STARTED TO BLOSSOM AND HAVE
MORE CONFIDENCE IN MYSELF! I
started taking pictures which before I
would hide._**

The thing that made me **_not give up_** was a
photo at a birthday party. My youngest
daughter was invited to a birthday POOL party.
Heck no I wasn't going to wear a swim suit! I
would just sit around the pool. I had on a big
black shirt and cute capri jeans. I also wore my
hair straight back then. Then it happen?
Picture time with the moms. Now I remember
looking at the other moms and thinking "she is
skinny, she is medium and she is about my
size. OK this picture won't be that bad, I have
been doing Zuuumbaaa. I was standing on the
outside with the moms, not in the middle
where you can hide. But when I was tagged on

FB and saw the picture for the first time, I freaked out. I untagged myself so fast. You'd of thought I just heard my lottery numbers. Running to grab my ticket to make sure I was not hearing things.

MY MOMENT

It was an awful feeling. I was bigger than everyone in that picture. I was so embarrassed because I felt like everyone saw and was laughing at me. I cried. That was my moment. I needed to try harder and change. I was not happy with what I looked like.

That moment is what kept me going. I kept going with what was working for me. I stopped eating candy, stopped drinking diet cokes and kept walking because I was changing my system. I lost almost a hundred pounds without going to the gym. Then I wanted definition. I WANTED to keep going. I was more confident and not even embarrassed to go the gym. The reason why I love to workout is because it is fun. I am just changing what I want. I am in control with what I put in my body and my mind isn't stressing out about losing weight. It's fun now.

Another thing I hear is "I don't have time." Don't get mad but YES you do. Do you have time to eat? Well there you go. You just need to change what you eat. Now "listen" I am not a cook and I still did it. There is a restaurant or fast food joint on every corner selling their food and you can change their food into your food. Get what you pay for. Later I did learn how to make my favorite low sugar treats because I wanted to. So can you! And if you are a cook, boy you could whip up so many great meals. You would benefit yourself more in the end.

So you have to change the way you eat, change your metabolism into a burning machine and have fun when you workout or walk. Take your glamour shots to remind you that you can do it. Strength is in your hands but willpower is in the mind.

Rule#5.
Quit Diet Cokes because first rule; this is not a diet.

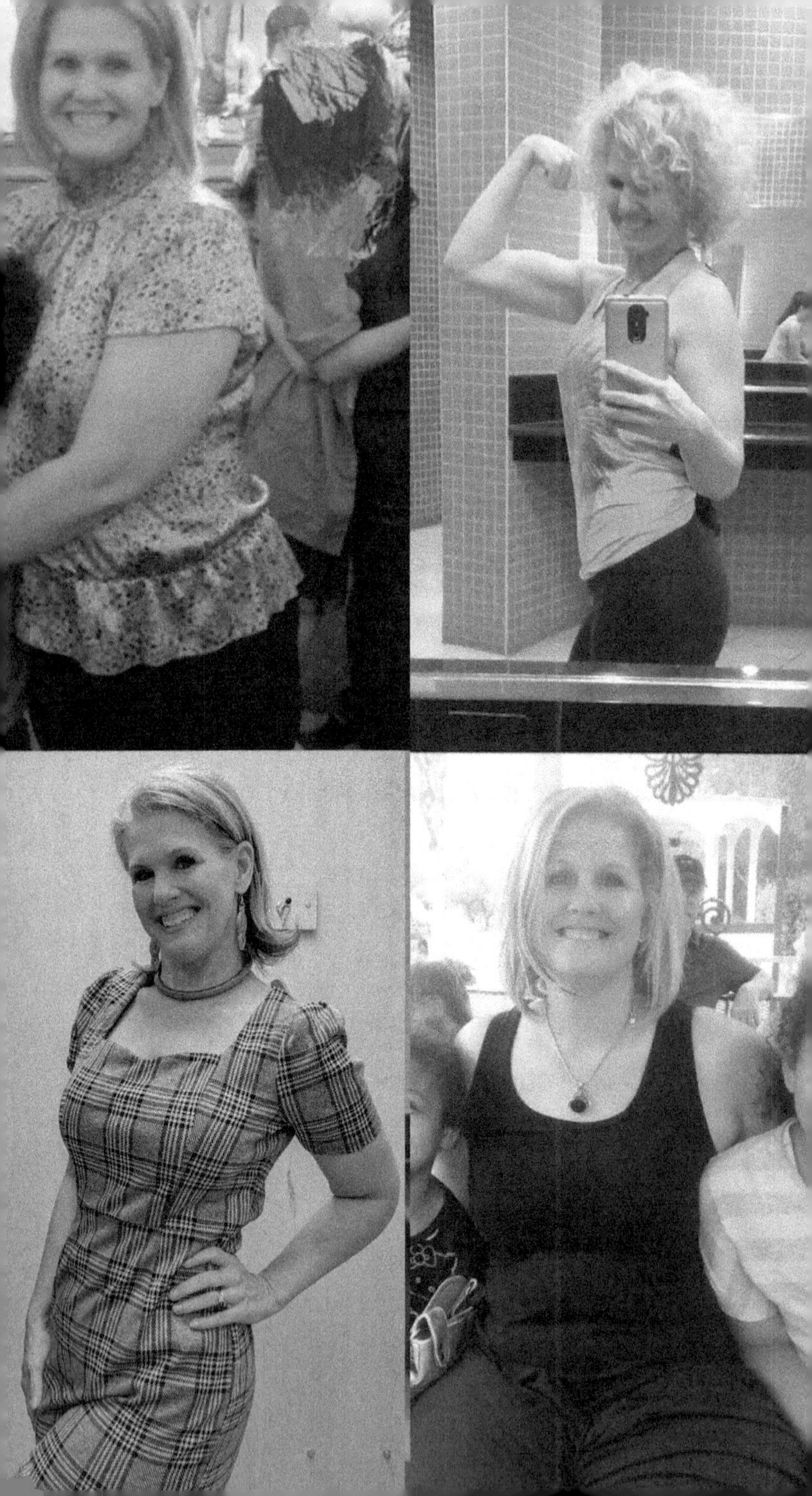

Seeing what you Accomplished
RULE#6

For me a glamour shot is what showed me my results more than people telling me I lost weight. I could see my results. It helped me keep going because I remember that moment of being the biggest one in the picture. Determination is the fire in your heart to keep you going. So if you do not have fun and enjoy your weight loss transformation, how is going to work? You won't want to keep going. You give up. Taking a photo of yourself when you've accomplished something is a good thing. You don't have to show it to anyone if you don't want to. It is just a reminder that you did the workout or you have the willpower to change what you did not like. That is why it is rule number six because sometimes you forget when your done. You forget when no one reminds you how big your were. You can look back and see you did it without anyone but yourself telling you. I DID IT!!

Rule#6.
Glamour Shots

I went shopping and tried on dresses because I did not want to do it before my weight loss.

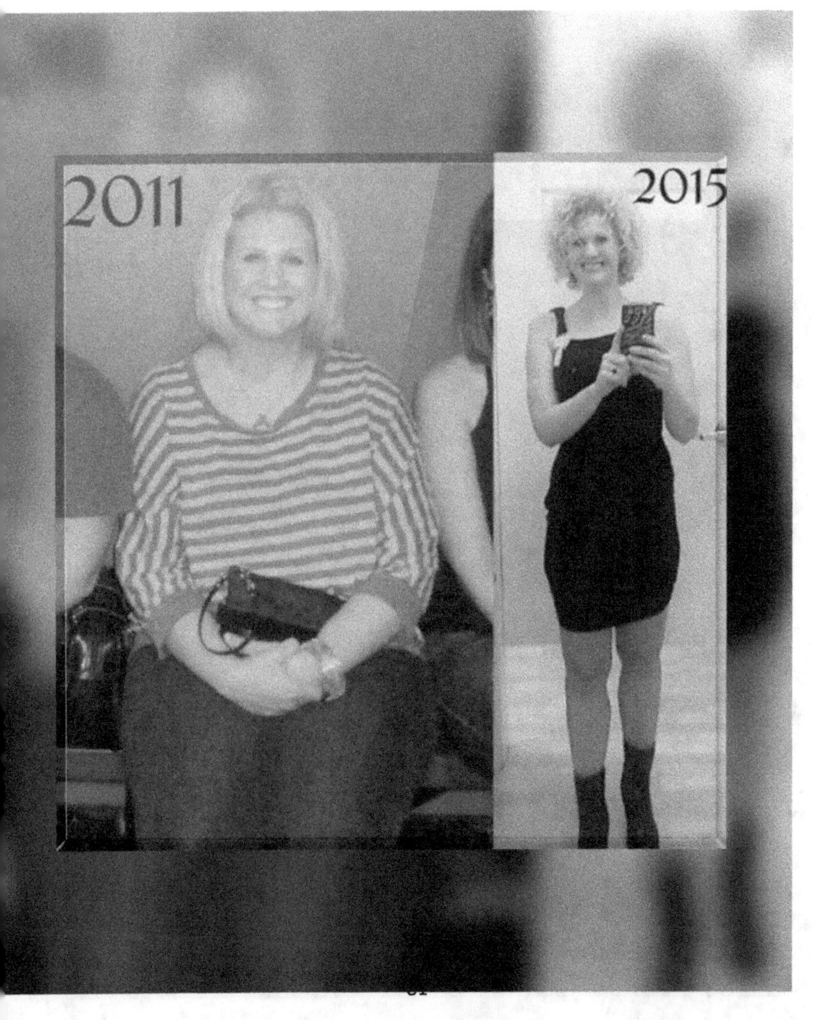

I hiked up a mountain and watched the sunrise. I wouldn't been able to that before my weight loss.

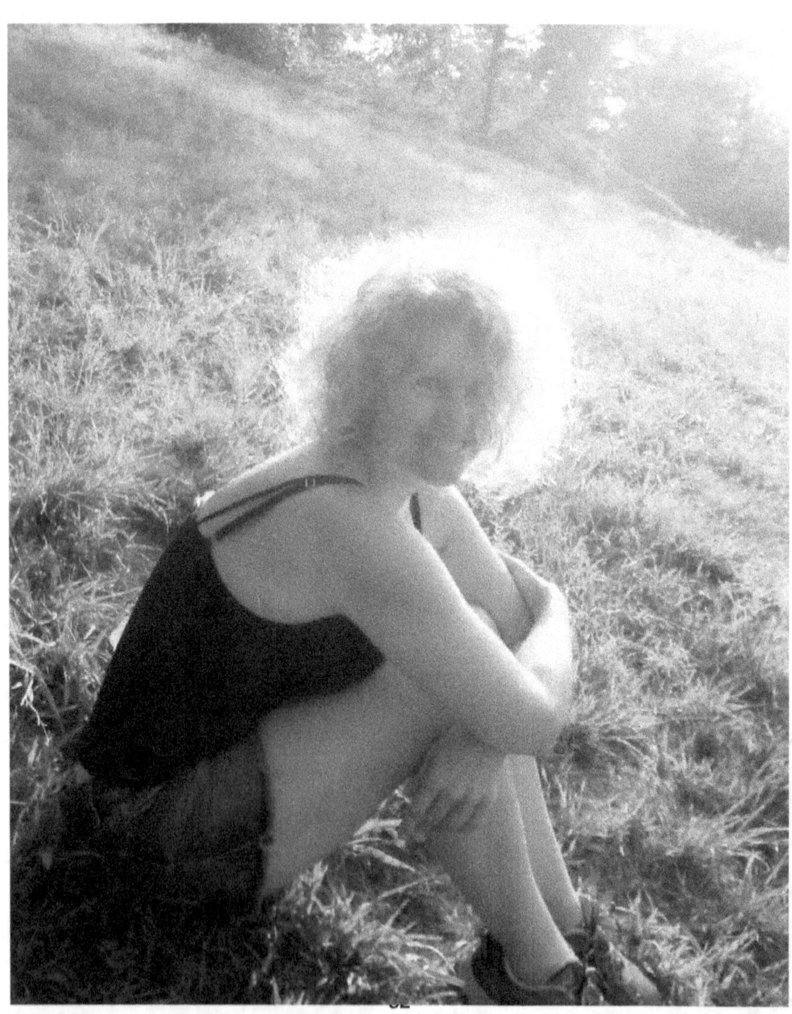

I broke down my wall and
now live the life I wanted to.

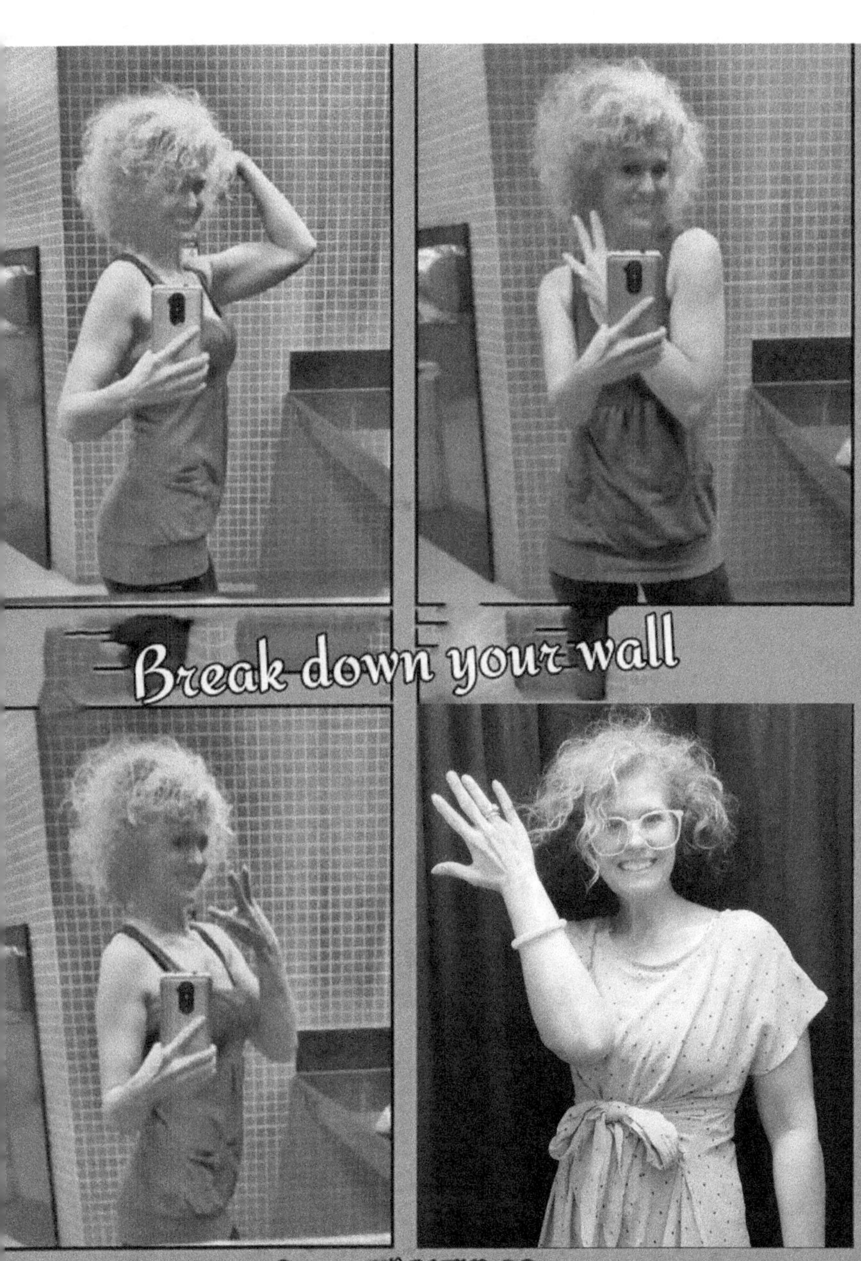

My Conclusion

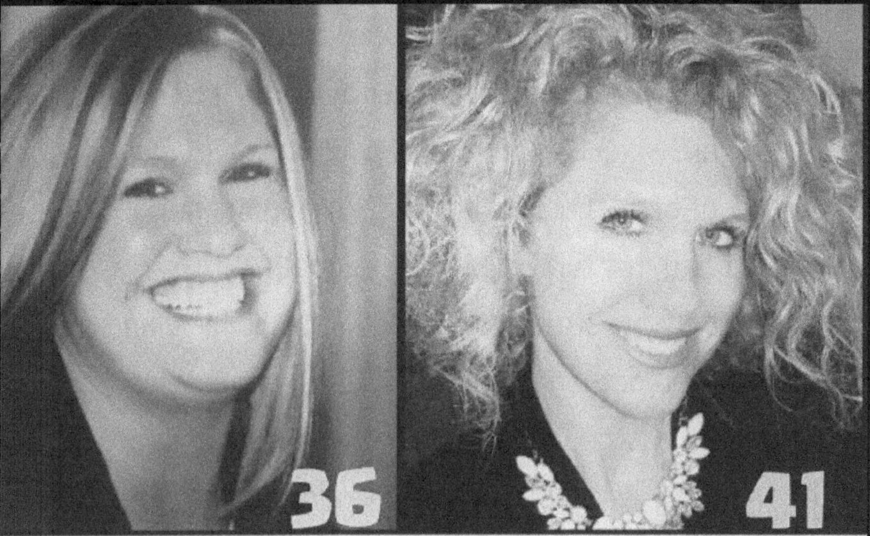

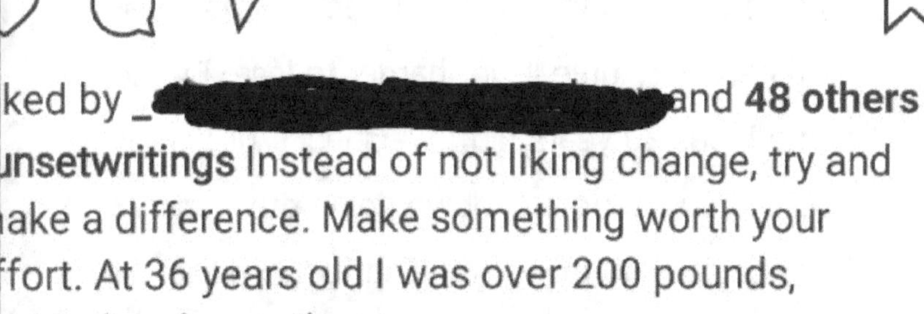

iew Insights

Promote

ked by _⬛⬛⬛ and **48 others**

unsetwritings Instead of not liking change, try and ake a difference. Make something worth your ffort. At 36 years old I was over 200 pounds, arried and a mother.

My conclusion is this. If you are in your 20's and say you can eat McDonald's everyday and not gain weight. Only time will tell. But most people can not eat a McDonald's hamburger and fries with a Dr. Pepper everyday and not gain weight. When I first graduated and moved out of my parents house, I started my first job. I had just turned 18 and weighed 145. Everyday after work I would stop at sonic and get a foot-long coney, chili cheese tater tots and a large Dr.Pepper. I gained 20 pounds within 4 months. It took me almost 5 months to loose the weight by starving myself. That was my first diet battle of ever being over weight. As soon as I started going back to my old eating routine I gained it back a little bit at a time. Every time it got harder to lose. By the time I was 30 years old I weighed 170. I went up and down, up and down doing the same diet of starving myself but I introduced Diet Soda into my life. Then I had my first child. I was up to 200 LBS. I lost 10 pounds after the first baby. Then I had my second child, I got up to 260 LBS. I lost 30 LBS after the second baby. I battled my with my 230 weight most of my 30's. The starving diet did not work any more or anything else I tried. Until I changed my system. I changed my routine to something I could live with. I believed I could do it and I did not give up. It is all in the mindset. If you believe it will happen, it will. ***The 6 Rules on Losing Weight*** is what got me through the change. I hope if you battle a roller coaster of diets this will help you succeed in who you want to look like when you look in the mirror and smile. Someone that conquered their battle of the diets.

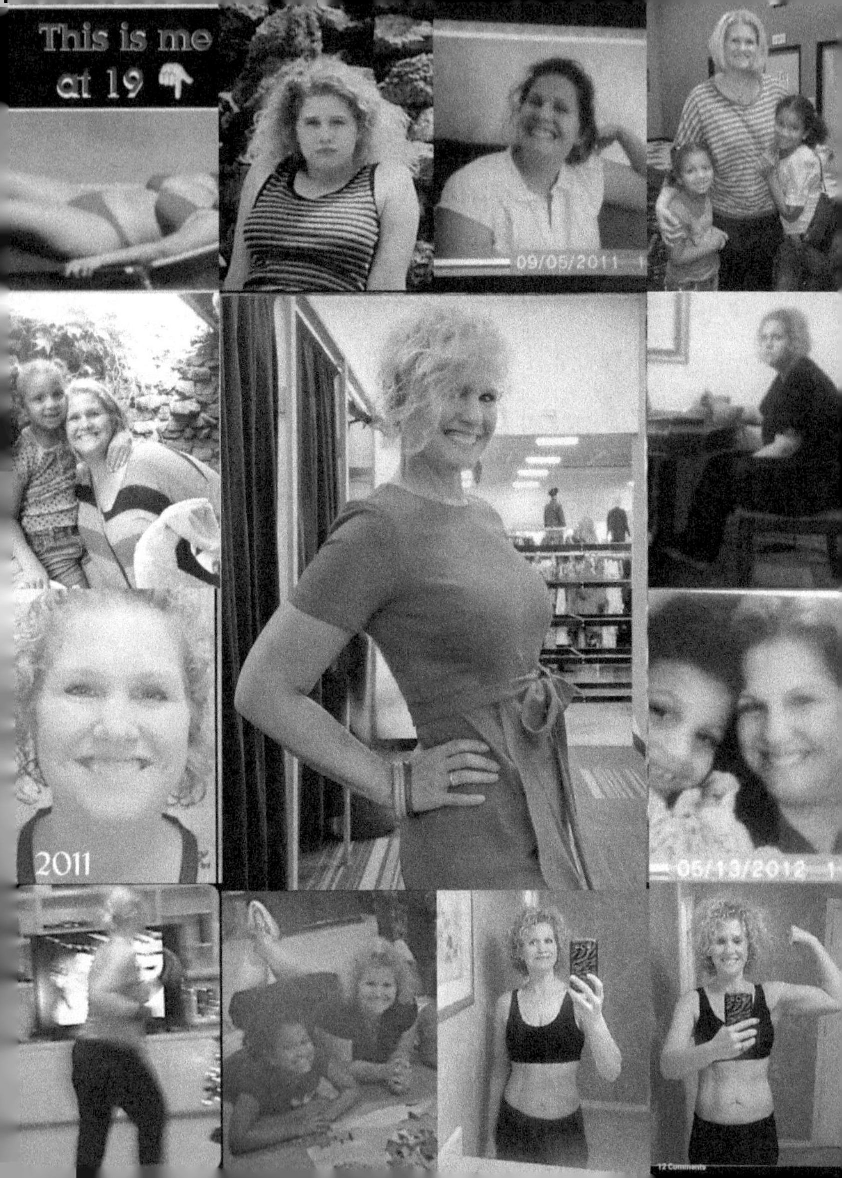

This is me
at 19
09/05/2011
2011
05/13/2012
12 Comments

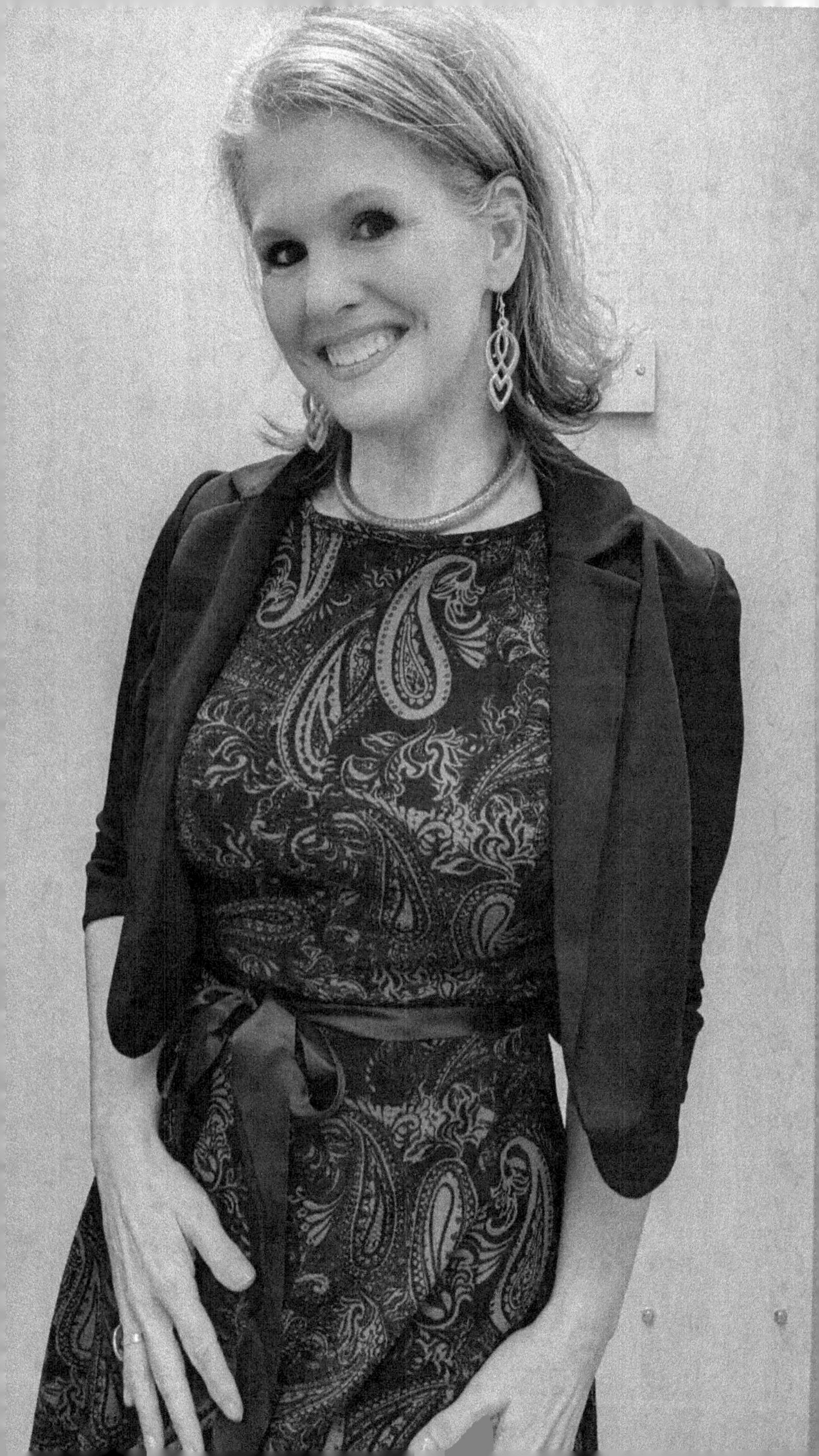

After I wrote this book in 2018, I created a product where you can take a hands free selfie. I took a lot of glamour shot photos but I did not like my phone in the photo. I broke down another wall in 2019. I created a material that is called Chriset Flex. It adheres to the back of your phone and then it can adhere to mirrors, glass, metal, ceramic, plastic and most flat surfaces. It is a reusable, removable stick. First, I created a phone facing, then into something better. I turned it into a real selfie sticker, then into a bracelet and jewelry. I created a combo of all these things.

The Halo Bracelet is something you can wear where ever you go and then you can use it to take a hands free selfie. The Real Selfie Sticker is something you can place on the back of your phone and take it where ever you go. This was one of my dreams and now it can go with this book. God is amazing and I could not of done any of this without him.

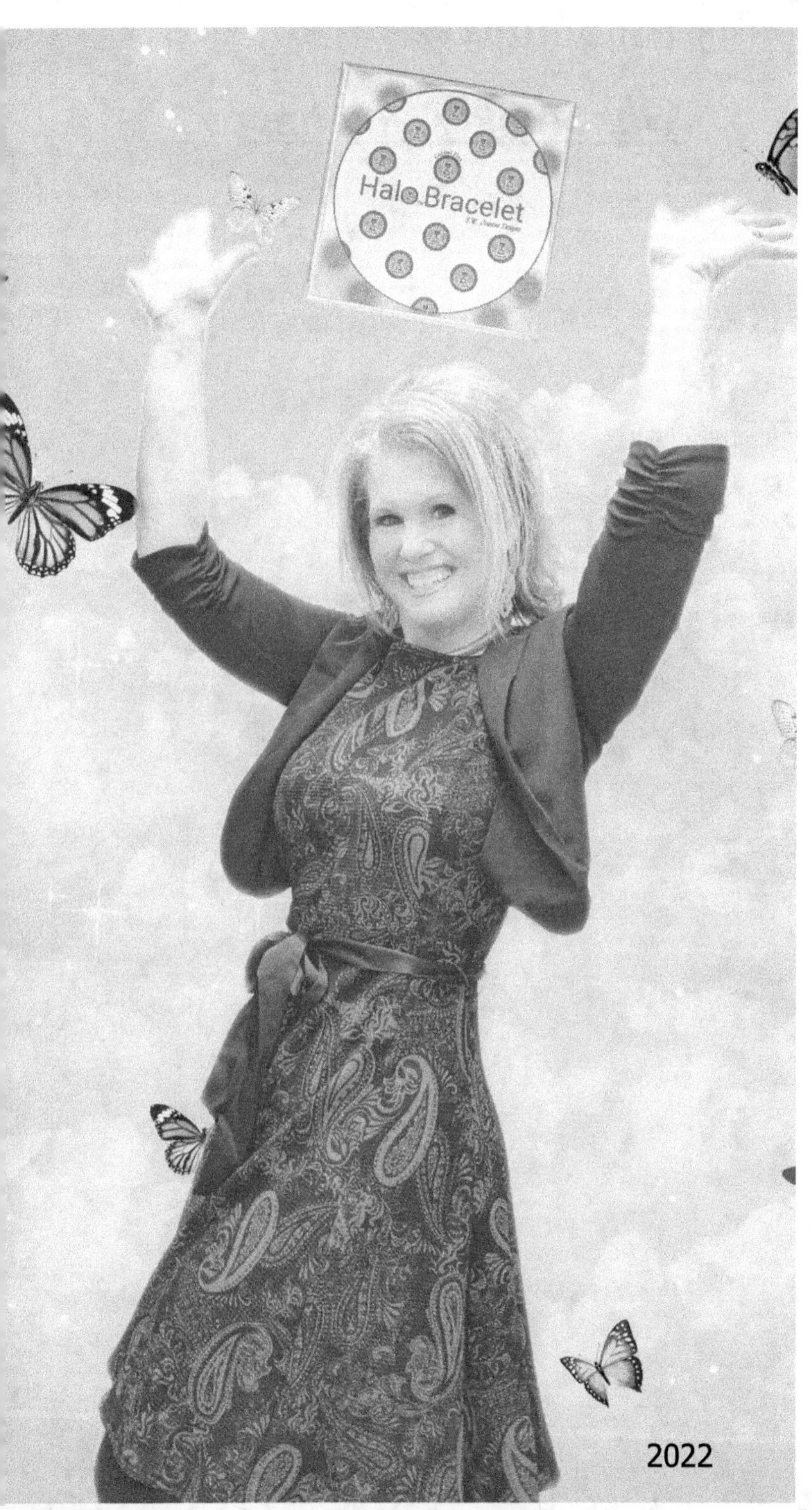

Halo Bracelet
2022

<u>What makes you happy?</u>

Goals and Accomplishments

Your wall

Dreams and Desires